The 5 Tibetan Rites For Beginners

Learn The Secret To Anti-Aging By Practicing The 5 Tibetan Rites

By Michele Gilbert

Visit My Amazon Author Page

Dedicated to those who choose to stretch beyond their own limits and to seek a more abundant and fulfilling life.

Your thoughts are creative.

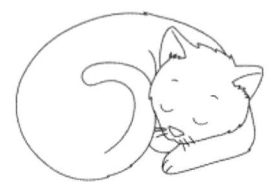

Michele Gilbert

My Free Gift To You!

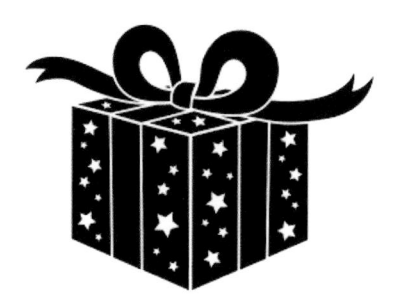

As a way of saying thank you for downloading my book, I am willing to give you access to a selected group of readers who (every week or so) receive inspiring, life-changing kindle books at deep discounts, and sometimes even absolutely free.

Wouldn't it be great to get amazing Kindle offers delivered directly to your inbox?

Wouldn't it be great to be the first to know when I'm releasing new fresh and above all sharply discounted content?

But why would I so something like this?

Why would I offer my books at such a low price and even give them away for free when they took me countless hours to produce?

Simple…. because I want to spread the word.!

For a few short days Amazon allows Kindle authors to promote their newly released books by offering them deeply discounted (up to 70% price discounts and even for free. This allows us to spread the word extremely quickly allowing users to download thousands and thousands of copies in a very short period of time.

Once the timeframe has passed, these books will revert back to their normal selling price. That's why you will benefit from being the first to know when they can be downloaded for free!

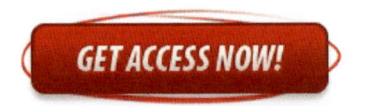

So are you ready to claim your weekly Kindle books?

You are just one click away! Follow the link below and sign up to start receiving awesome content

Thank you and Enjoy!

Table of contents

My Free Gift To You!

Introduction

Finding the Rites

The History of the Rites

The Five Tibetan Rites of Rejuvenation

Tibetan Idea of Healing

Conclusion

Preview of My New Book

My Free Gift To You!

About Michele

Introduction

In the Western world there is nothing my mysterious and more confusing to our Western sensibilities and culture than that of the East, especially when it comes to religious practices. In fact, there are so many people in the West that don't really have a firm grasp on what it means to be Buddhist, a Taoist, a Confucian, or any of the other Eastern Philosophies that populate the world. Outside of the ideals of Christianity and the myriad of practices that spawned from the formation of that faith, most of us don't even have a clue what it's all about.

In fact, I'd go so far to say that there are plenty of people practicing Eastern Philosophies that have approached it with a rather New Age flippancy that is usually reserved for buffet lines. Most pick and choose the ideals, tenants, or practices that serve them best and fold it into their custom made faith. Regardless of the approach's effectiveness, reverence, or blasphemy, the result is usually the same. There is a haphazard nature to this approach and there are so many who are looking for more to add to it.

But, perhaps you're not looking for a new spiritual practice that you want to incorporate into your own doctrine or worship method. Perhaps you've heard about the miraculous benefits of something called the Five Tibetan Rites. This is the mystical and strange practice that has been performed for over 2,500 years by the monks of Tibet. It is the spiritual practice that has been reported to invigorate, heal, and calm the body in ways that no other practice can. Whether this is true or not remains a matter of debate. However, the Five Tibetan Rites are a mystery to most people and very few actually know of their existence.

This is the very essence of arcane knowledge. This is what so many people desire and hunger for and I'm going to give you all the information that you're going to need to know about the Five Tibetan Rites. Whether you're a devout, practitioner of the Easter Philosophies, or you're just curious, I'm going to give you all the information that will be of help to you in understanding and mastering this practice for yourself.

So, let's get to work understanding what the Five Tibetan Rites actually are and what they mean to you.

Finding the Rites

The past is a fickle and cruel thing in parts of the world. While the sands of time continue to flow, reverence, importance, and value is often subjective to the whims of the ruling power or the populace of the times. In the 1950's the Chinese Government invaded the Tibetan Plateau and caused massive widespread damage, the effects of which are still being felt today and will be felt for ages to come. The Chinese were so destructive and so violent toward the Tibetan people that we are extremely luck that an entire culture and way of life was not radically extinguished by the Chinese Government.

When the Chinese invaded, Tibet was known as a religious territory, a land of faith and contemplation. It was one of the most densely populated places on the planet for holy sites, devout monks, and pacifists. Prior to the invasion 6,259 monasteries, convents, and holy sites existed in Tibet unharmed and in pristine condition as they had been for thousands of years. When the Chinese government was finished with their invasion only eight locations remained undestroyed. This doesn't mean that some were simply shot at, like propaganda would have the world believe. These locations were leveled and destroyed.

While countless pieces of priceless artifacts, spiritual texts, and historical records were lost in the destruction and the violence, but hope endures. There were many researchers still in the area and black market deals were utilized through a network of renegade Tibetans, underground monks, and criminal avenues that were employed to get some of the information out of the country. Not only were some pieces of the Tibetan history salvaged, but there were many other monasteries in the Himalayas that contained information about many of the Tibetan rituals, customs, and culture.

One of the salvaged pieces of information was something known as the Five Tibetan Rites of Rejuvenation. The story around the Five Tibetan Rites is something ripped straight from the pages of an adventure novel and is quite fascinating. While many people have worked in translation detail trying to piece together what information we have from Tibetan and Indian texts, the majority of the information that they accumulated references the Rites existing back 2,500 years. However, their work was fairly limited being compared to the works of an antiquarian book dealer known as Jerry Watt.

Jerry Watt is the man who decided that combing through the pieces of information that was destroyed in the Chinese assault on the Tibetan Plateau was not going to recover anything substantial. Any information that had been salvaged by this network of renegades and criminals was now being snatched up on the black market by criminals and collectors from all over the world. No, if he wanted to find something of substance, he was going to need to look elsewhere. So, like many historians before him, Jerry went looking to one of the most destructive forces on the planet and that is the history of the British Empire.

The British Empire spanned from their small portion of their island in the Atlantic coast of Europe to dominating the largest empire in the history of the world. Unlike the destructive force of the Chinese Government that had raided and destroyed so much in Tibet, the British were fascinated by their conquered subjects. When the British army invaded a territory, nation, or kingdom, when the army had stabilized the area, merchants and scholars flooded the area to report back to London what had been acquired by the Empire. As a result, every subject on the planet seems to have had some sort of covering by a British academic who took to the field for an adventure to write a book, pamphlet, or paper on the material that fascinated them.

What Jerry Watts eventually discovered was a man named Peter Kelder. As of right now, Peter Kelder is the only man in the history of the world who seems to have met someone who had personal contact with the practitioners of these Rites. He's an indirect witness to these practices and is our best source of information. While there are disputes upon the legitimacy of the booklet Kelder wrote, it has yet to receive any substantial blow to destroy its reputation and credibility among researchers and spiritual experts alike. There was nothing that could be more thrilling than arriving in India and searching for knowledge and information about the supernatural, occult, and bizarre.

At the time, there's something that captivated London and the British Empire about the mystical and the occult world. Christianity was beginning to lose its control and the mystical, pagan, and bizarre had started to infect the people of England and many other elite European cities. So any curiosities that could be recovered, found, or researched were in high demand. This led Jerry Watt to find a man referenced in his papers as Colonel Bradford. Colonel Bradford is an alias and not the man's real name.

Colonel Bradford had heard legends of monks in the Himalayas that had found a sort of Fountain of Youth that had given them immense power to survive for years without aging. The legends of these monks were whispered in the shadows and passed from source to source until Colonel Bradford decided that he wanted to see if there was any truth to the legends that he was hearing. So, heading in to the mountains, Colonel Bradford found himself in the lamasery where they taught him something that captivated the world for centuries.

Known as the Five Tibetan Rites of Rejuvenation, these rituals and practices were shown to him and explained thoroughly while he was living with the lamas in the lamasery. In the end, when Colonel Bradford left them, he brought with them secret knowledge that he delivered to Kelder in the form of his booklet. These skills and practices were highly wrapped up in the beliefs of the lamasery and remained fairly discarded and hidden for a long period of time before it was brought to light and seen of interest. Kelder's booklet became the touchstone to ancient knowledge that has left people baffled and enthralled for years since and it is one of the best-kept secrets in the world.

While the history of how the Five Tibetan Rites of Rejuvenation is perhaps one of the most fascinating tales in the history of searching for lost literature, but it was actually found that truly proves to be one of the most intriguing and exciting pieces of information that we have. As far as the spiritual community is concerned, the Five Tibetan Rites of Rejuvenation holds the secrets of the world. It's one of the most intriguing questions that have captivated the world. How do you evade the passage of time? Can a single person live indefinitely? As far as the lamas of the mysterious lamasery in the Himalayas are concerned, there's a way. Not only is there a way to stay young forever, but they're strangely simple for you to partake in on a daily basis.

So, how are you going to find this fountain of youth? Well, by reading this book, I'm going to give you a glimpse inside the world of the Five Tibetan Rites of Rejuvenation. Now let's get started on the path to eternal youth.

The History of the Rites

Now that you know the history of the booklet, it's time to have a chat about the actual history of the actions that you're going to be taking part in. There's a lengthy history you need to be aware of that I'm going to make simple and understanding for you in a way that doesn't make you feel like you've just read a textbook.

Why is a history necessary? Well, because in the matter of spiritual disciplines and skills, you need to understand what is actually happening to you. This isn't something you can just slap on your life and expect yourself to be able to tap into spiritual power. While spirituality is open and available to anyone, there is a strange sort of belief in the world today that spiritual matters can just be picked up or chosen at will without doing any of the necessary preparation, due diligence, or discipline that is required to truly make the spiritual matters a part of your life. So, to better understand what it is you're doing, then you need to actually know why you're doing it, how these skills are going to help you, and why you need to take part of it in your life. After all, once you know about something that can genuinely reverse your aging, according to legend, then wouldn't you want to make sure that you utilize it accurately and that you know what it is you're doing? You want this to actually work after all. So, why should you care about this lamasery, what they have to say and why they might actually know what it is they're talking about? So, in order to understand why these are all important, we need to explore the history of it.

In order to properly understand what it is that these lamas believed, you need to understand that there is a strong tie between Buddhism and Hinduism, in fact, much like Christianity is born out of the tenants of Judaism, so too is Buddhism born out of Hinduism. The tenants of Hinduism share a lot of the basic spiritual disciplines of Buddhism, but in the end, that can all be traced back to the Buddha who gave birth to the Buddhism.

The history of the Buddha essentially comes down to a prince who was born to a privileged and lavished lifestyle at the height of war and civil strife in India, all of which was born within the animosity of the caste system and warring states. When he looked around and saw all of this death and suffering in the world, he decided to abandon the world that he had been born into. He cast off the world of beautiful women, riches, amazing food, and the finest materials that he could ever want or desire. By getting rid of all of these, the Buddha began an adventure to discover what was truly important in life, how to get rid of all the evil in his life, and ultimately, to find out what his purpose and position in the chaos of the world truly was.

In order to do this, he abandoned everything and inevitably discovered what it was that he considered the secret to all suffering in the world. The idea that desire alone dictated the evils of the world and that abstaining from the things you desired and by rewriting the thoughts, actions, and beliefs of your life, you can free yourself, was a revolutionary thought that changed his whole life. In a world of shamen, yogis, and Hindu priests all believing in a predestination of our existence, the power of psychic energy, and the existence of gods and demons, Buddha said that it ultimately didn't matter on a personal, pragmatic sense as far as spirituality was concerned. To him, a man or woman needed only to erase desire from their life and they could find that everything that was evil or harmful in their life could be removed. This was a radical and strange idea that was hard to convince people of at first, but eventually, Buddhism began to spread.

Wherever Buddhism spread, it was not immune or invulnerable to the same problems that face every other religion in the world. As it spread, old faiths of the region began to meld together with the old customs that were serviced as metaphors to the new faith inevitably began to bleed together. As Buddhism spread across India, it picked up practices of the Yogis and Hindus. Crawling over the Himalayas, Buddhism came head to head with the Tao and Confucius in the coming years, but the true epitome of Buddhism's monastic society was based in the Himalayas and on the northern plateau of Tibet. In these areas, it became a vortex of religious beliefs, all of the monks sought truth in the faiths that were washing over the land, tying together the threads of truth that they found among each of them.

What these monks inevitably developed and found was a pure form of faith that was developed upon the tenants of Buddhism, but was expanded upon the questioning of everything. They sought answers, but also acknowledged the truth that was found in the questions as well. Among all of these, they collected immense amounts of information that we might construe as mystical or questionable, but numerous eyewitness accounts question the doubt many of us have. In fact, it demands answers on the part of the doubter.

Essentially, the spiritual history of the Himalayas and the Tibetan Plateau are mixed with a melting pot of faiths, beliefs, and systems that have churned across Asia over the centuries. Of course, this melting pot is genuinely a pot forged out of the ideals and tenants of Buddhism. While you may see similarities with the Five Tibetan Rites and Yoga, you'll find that it's still practiced with the ideals of Buddhism at the heart of it.

So, if you want to know even more about what it was that these monks found to be truthful and the source of spiritual power, then you really need to dive into what it is Buddhism wants for you in your life. It's a vast and intriguing faith that is based upon Eight Steps that you'll be applying to your life in order to govern your thoughts and actions in a more successful way for you and the world around you. It's very interesting and a very unique faith that I would strongly recommend that you take a look at, even if you're a firm believer in another faith. It never hurts to see what it is that others believe in and how similar so many faiths truly are. After all, the core of goodness and morality isn't that vast or unique when it comes to the faiths of the world. It's a great topic to discover and I highly recommend you look into it, especially if you're looking to apply these Five Tibetan Rites of Rejuvenation to your life.

Now, the fact that you know that the lamas in the lamasery that Colonel Bradford was visiting were collectors of knowledge and information pertaining to spiritual matters and had strong influences in Hinduism, Yoga, and predominantly Buddhism, you'll understand why these Rites feel a lot more like you're practicing yoga than you're practicing a Buddhist discipline. Now, without any further history lessons, let's actually get down to the brass tacks of what these Five Tibetan Rites of Rejuvenation truly are.

The Five Tibetan Rites of Rejuvenation

Now, without further adieu, let's get into the Five Tibetan Rites of Rejuvenation. These are the ancient techniques that are going to help you change your life and regress the effects of aging and to add somewhere around ten years to your life, if the legends are to be taken as truth. Of course, since I'm not able to compare my own utilization of these habits with the length of my life with and without them, I can't tell you with one hundred percent truth and accuracy, I will tell you that I feel great while I've been doing them. You do feel a sort of inner peace and boiling energy under the skin. You're going to love it.

But, before we get started, the lamasery taught Colonel Bradford that there are seven points of psychic energy that are responsible for the aging process and the sole reason for why your body is either not feeling well or why you're breaking down. As far as they believe, these psychic vortexes are churning extremely fast throughout your younger years in your life and that when you get older they begin to slow. When these psychic vortexes begin to slow your body begins to decay, cellular regeneration, blood flow, and everything else begins to slow, even the elasticity of the skin. The only way to stop this inevitable decay that leads to death, you have to find a way to get these vortexes to start flowing faster and to stop the slowing process. Thus, the Five Rites were developed to get these Five Rites churning and spinning as quickly as possible.

The real question that you probably have right now is where are these vortexes located? To answer that question, the monks spent years meditating and seeking out the best understanding of auras and the psychic flow of energy through the body to come to the ultimate conclusion that these vortexes number seven strong and that they're not exactly where you'd think they were.

The first vortex that you're going to find is located in the forehead in the pineal gland. The second vortex is found at the posterior part of the brain known as the pituitary gland. It's small, about the size of a pea and is at the base of the brain. The third vortex is in the neck, just above your collarbones and might actually be considered the throat, depends upon who you're talking to. Vortex number four is located in your liver. The fifth vortex is found in your sex glands, so either you're testicles or your ovaries. The final too vortexes are located in both of your knees, which are strong locations for grounding your spiritual energy. These are the locations of your vortexes and these are the locations that are going to be affected most by the actions of your Five Tibetan Rites of Rejuvenation.

Now, let's have a chat about the first rite that you're going to perform. With your arms outstretched from your shoulders, you're going to want to spin by turning from left to right until you're slightly dizzy. Does this sound and look silly? Yes, but you're getting your several of your vortexes stimulated by this action and you're getting them activated through this action.

Now, between each of these rites, it's important that you stand straight and just take a few breaths. Now, there are a lot of works and papers written about the importance of breathing with these rites, but one thing that leads many to find speculation with these claims is the simple fact that Colonel Bradford made no mention of this in his reports to Kelder, which would have been a not of importance to him. After all, the British were academics and they were extremely interested in the peculiarities and strangeness of these rituals, so if breathing was involved, Colonel Bradford made no mention of it after living in the lamasery with the lamas for a long duration of time. So, what I gather from this is that it wasn't of importance is simply the application of current meditation techniques to the old skills. Will breathing techniques hurt or hinder the results? I highly doubt it and if you feel the need to look into breathing techniques between these rites to better focus your energy, so be it. However, I want you to know that it doesn't seem very necessary to most academics on the matter.

The second rite is going to require you lay down on a rug and place your hands flat on the sides of your hips. Your fingers and palms flat on the floor with them slightly pointed toward each other. With your feet, you're going to want to pull them up with your legs straight as possible. Think of it as a sort of reverse crunch that is going to be activating your core. Lift your legs up ninety degrees and then keep pushing with your legs to be closer to your head. When you've finally hit the apex of your flexibility, then slowly lower your legs and make sure that you're keeping it in a controlled, flowing motion. You should repeat this exercise until you can feel the energy flowing through you. However, I know a lot of people who interpret that statement as doing it until they're exhausted. No, don't do it until you're exhausted, rather do it until you feel your energy flowing. This should never take longer than five minutes and five minutes is a very long time for you to be performing this rite. Again, when you're done, stand up, take a few breaths, and get yourself centered for the next rite.

The third rite is going to require that you knee down on the rug. When you're kneeling on the rug, place your hands on the front of your thighs and lean forward, curling your head forward so that your chin is touching your chest. When you've accomplished that, slide your hands to your butt cheeks or the backs of your thighs and lean backwards, opening up your chest and leaning your head back as far as you can. Don't go so far that it's painful, but make sure that you're opening up your body. Then lean yourself forward so that you're at the starting position again and repeat the exercise until you've reached a similar state that feels energized and motivated to move forward. Again, there's a moment where you should take your opportunity to stand up again and practice your controlled breathing to center yourself one more time. Once you've finished with the standing and breathing, it's time to move on to the next rite.

The fourth rite requires that you sit down with your back straight and your legs stretched out in front of you. Placing your hands along your sides, you should put your palms and fingers flat on the ground next to you, then digging the balls of your feet into the ground, dive your strength deep and push yourself up, so that your knees are bent. Your thighs, hips, and torso should all be flat without any arc or bend in your body. You should be supporting yourself with your feet, calves, hands and arms, all of them straight down. Hold yourself in this position for a moment before you slowly lower yourself back to the original position and continue to build a flow of energy and feel it empowering your body. This is probably the hardest rite to start out with and it's difficult to get a controlled flow going with your body when you're starting out. This is fine, but it's important that you build up your strength with this exercise and that posture is focused on. You want the flow to be fluid and strong. If you're shaking or jerking, it's going to affect the results of this rite. So, keep at it, build up your strength and do the best that you possibly can with it. Like always, when you're done with the set, stand up straight with great posture, feel the energy flowing around and through you as you breathe. Then, it's time to move on to the next set for you.

The final rite is going to be familiar to yoga experts as downward facing dog that flows into cobra position. Start out with your hands and your feet as your foundation, pushing up with your hips so that you bend into a triangle. It's extremely important for your posture that your legs are straight and that your arms and torso form a straight line bending from your hips downward. This is called downward facing dog in the yoga world. From here, you're going to want to push downward, controlling the motion with your warms so that your body forms a plank with your torso facing upward and your head leaning back. This is called the cobra position. For a more visual interpretation, I suggest that you actually look up the images to get a better idea. It's a basic move that doesn't require a whole lot of work and finesse in the yoga world, so I'm sure you'll be able to take care of it. Continue to build a flow with these positions and postures until you've hit the point where you feel like you've found the perfect energy flowing through your body.

When you're done with the final rite, stand up and breathe, feel your body relaxing and the energy flowing through you. By the time you're at the end of it, then you should be feeling an energy running through you and the invigoration is something you're going to really feel all around you. You have completed the Five Tibetan Rites of Rejuvenation that are going to flow through your body, revitalizing your seven vortexes and giving you a source of prolonged youthfulness. This isn't just energy so that you feel young, there is an actual physiological effect here that thousands of people have witnessed or experienced for themselves.

The final note that I should be mentioning is the fact that there are some who claim that there is a sixth rite. Now, before I tell you what the sixth rite is, I want to be completely upfront with you about the legitimacy of this rite. I'm not sure that I personally buy it. Again, there are a lot of speculation as to whether or not Kelder's book is legitimate or completely accurate about the world Colonel Bradford witnessed and experienced in the lamasery. Again, I want to stress the level of detail that the British academics at the time were accustomed to giving precedence to. If Kelder's book is not complete with the details that were important, then I would stress that the book be taken entirely as false. The authenticity of this book cannot be picked apart. Either it is entirely accurate or entirely false. To claim that it is incomplete would imply that the lamas at Bradford's lamasery were both withholding information and deceiving him, or that contemporaries know better. I'm inclined to doubt in both of those facts. But, there are many contemporaries that believe there is a sixth rite. Take it or leave it according to your convictions.

The sixth rite is essentially going to be a moment where you sit down, meditate and practice several ritual breathing techniques. Now, if this is just a meditation exercise, then I would suggest that you take it at that. Meditation has many amazing qualities to it and there isn't a religion in the world that doesn't practice it as a spiritual discipline. But, I would simply take it as a meditation practice at the end of the Five Tibetan Rites of Rejuvenation and leave it at that. I wouldn't actually incorporate it into the actual practices.

Now, these are the Five Tibetan Rites of Rejuvenation in their complete essence with a sixth added on if you take the word of some contemporaries. Again, take it or leave it depending upon what you believe. However, the Five Rites are famous for their qualities and their powers with those who practice them. It is strongly suggested that you practice the Five Rites at least once a day to ensure that your vortexes are flowing with energy and strongly empowered. There are many people who make sure that they do the Five Rites on multiple occasions throughout the day, especially when they're feeling tired or like there's an energy lull that is hitting them.

The great thing about the Five Tibetan Rites of Rejuvenation is the fact that they're not going to take up enormous amounts of time. In fact, they're going to take up around twenty minutes of your time when you practice them. It shouldn't take you more than twenty minutes for you to complete the rites on their own. You can enfold them into your life whenever you have time for them. So if you're not a morning person, then you're going to find that you can work them in at the end of the day or during a break at the office. Whenever you need to fit them in, you'll be able to. The only reason you won't be able to incorporate them into your life is that you're actively not making time for them. So there's really no excuse for you to take twenty minutes to vitalize your body.

Now, the final aspect that I want to stress to you is the value of healing as perceived by the Tibetan people and the monks living in the monasteries and lamaseries. So, let's have a quick look at why they believe that these rites are going to change your life for the better.

Tibetan Idea of Healing

Buddhism is an extremely cognizant and mental faith that requires that you spend the majority of your time changing the ways you think, perceive, and experience the world around you. This is essentially the battle and the struggle that every Buddhist must fight throughout their life. It is the process of removing yourself from any equation that you might face in your life. You need to remove any selfishness, desire, or value on yourself and place it in the world around you. This is a difficult struggle and it's something that requires immense amounts of dedication and work in your life.

From this value, it is believed that if you have the values of your life in the right spot, then your mind will be a healthy place of power and energy in your life that will ultimately fuel your body into a healthy and harmonious place that cannot be torn down. It is believed that those who spend hours meditating and training their minds, their bodies will follow suit.

This is something that many people in the medical field point to today, although they're not directly pointing to Buddhism, they do sight the idea as a basic core. It's the idea that a positive and healthy mind is going to stimulate growth and development where a negative mind is going to hinder and decay the human body so that it doesn't recover from the damages that the body suffers from. So, the application of a healthy mind is incredibly invaluable. This is a vital part of the Five Tibetan Rites of Rejuvenation.

You cannot separate the Tibetan idea of healing from the Rites that you've been shown in this book. You have to be willing to dedicate a substantial amount of time to your mental health if you expect your body to have the same amount of durability, growth, and vitality that we're all seeking from this fountain of youth.

This isn't demanding that you become Mister or Miss Sunshine with the snap of a finger, but it does require that you start to take action and not in a superficial sense. If you want to have a positive change in your mental health, then you need to acknowledge suffering, understand the root source of it, and then focus on how it can be altered or challenged for the better. The goal isn't to run away from suffering, but to understand that suffering is inevitable in this world and that through your actions you can relieve it, stop it, or redirect the suffering into a positive energy that can be utilized for the betterment of humanity. Remember, take yourself out of the equation and utilize yourself as a force of good in the world. That's the key to all of this. Then, when you perform the Five Tibetan Rites of Rejuvenation, you're not seeking this flow of immortality for your own selfish desires, but to actually help the world around you.

Do some good with the power you've been given and have the right mindset. These are going to be the keys to the success of your time with the Five Tibetan Rites of Rejuvenation. So, you understand that this isn't just a ritual that you can pick up and master, you actually have to practice and tap into the knowledge that the Buddhist monks and lamas discovered and have dedicated their lives to understanding and implementing.

Conclusion

We live in a world where it's very vogue to pick up parts of spirituality, morality, and religion and kind of then construct your own emotional or spiritual paradigm to follow and dedicate your life to. While this might be an interesting and fun way to approach spirituality in the world, it often waters down or takes away the power required for some really interesting and powerful spiritual beliefs to take effect in the lives of those who practice them. I hope that in this book, I have given you enough history, background, and spiritual implementation for the Five Tibetan Rites of Rejuvenation to take part in your life and to really develop them as part of your life.

In this book, we have recounted the amazing and extremely complex history of finding the Five Tibetan Rites of Rejuvenation. It is a history worthy of its own adventure movie and it is quite possibly one of the most fortunate discoveries in the history of the world, especially in Buddhist literature. Next, we talked about how the history of Buddhism is filled with a drive to discover and find the truth in a world that was full of churning spiritual ideas, and how they incorporated the truths they discovered into their understanding of the world around them. Next, I taught you the Five Tibetan Rites of Rejuvenation and showed you how simple it was for you to incorporate them into your life on a daily basis. Next, you can find the Buddhist ideas of healing as interpreted by the Tibetan monks.

Overall, I hope that you found what you were looking for in this book and that you can now implement the Five Tibetan Rites of Rejuvenation as part of your life. I wish you good luck and hope that these help you in the future as you explore the world and where you fit into it now.

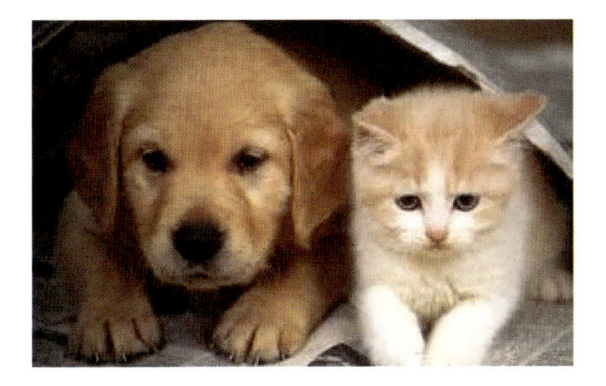

Before you go, I'd like to say thank you for purchasing my book.

I know you could have picked so many other books to read .But you took a chance on me.

So A Big thanks for downloading this book and reading it all the way to completion.

Now I would like to ask a *small* favor.

Could you please take a minute or two to leave a review for this book on Amazon?

Click here

The feedback will help me continue to publish more kindle books that will help people to get better results in their lives.

And if you found it helpful in anyway then please let me know :-)

Preview of My New Book

[Wicca: The Ultimate Beginners Guide For Witches and Warlocks: Learn Wicca Magic Spells, Traditions and Rituals](#)

What is Wicca?

So you're interested in Wicca, or maybe you've already started your adventure into the big world of one of the oldest religions in the world. It's a noble quest, as is the pursuit of higher knowledge in any religion. For you to continue your journey, or perhaps to start it, you're going to need to begin somewhere and reading is always the best place to start. So here you go.

To be honest, Wicca has, like every religion, evolved over the long years that it has existed. What started as blind paganism and mysticism has adapted and evolved, tearing apart the cruel ambition, dark rituals, and bloody rites that gave it a sense of barbarism. What is left is the enlightened, adapted version of the old ways that have been passed down for ages. Like most religions, there are sects and factions, all of which have ideological differences that distinguish them. But for a brief history on the faith, I will be your esteemed guide through history.

Let's start at the beginning:

In the early twentieth century, the idea of Wicca was first born. Yes, we do trace our roots all the way back to the foundations of religion itself and it is often said that we are one of the oldest faiths because of this. However, to be quite honest, so do most religions. Wicca itself was founded by the meeting of clandestine groups that some call covens. Wait, let me clarify, we call them covens. Our faith existed in silence and in secrecy due to Christian persecution. Originating mostly from European traditions and resurgence in the mystic arts, it wasn't until the Fifties that we were actually given the name the Craft. This was really the capitalistic boom of our religion, which, from my own personal beliefs, is one of our darker periods. We were much more interested in popularity and attention rather than the pursuit of the Craft.

What you are stepping into now is a much different faith than was previously established in the Sixties and the Seventies after the sensational blossom of our beliefs in the Fifties took root. Today, most Wicca practitioners that you meet are quietly dedicated to the faith and beliefs that they have been taught. Though there are many covens in the world today, meeting and practicing, it is a deeply personalized faith that we follow and it is dedicated to a lot of independent research and development.

Here's what we do not do, or at least to the best of my knowledge. We do not eat babies, we do not worship the devil, and we do not offer human sacrifices. Like I have said before, our faith is extremely popularized by society, no thanks to some of our own members.

Honestly, if you were to meet an average Wiccan on the streets, you probably wouldn't know it. Sure, we draw an element of society, the lost souls, the searching, and the misunderstood. We welcome them and we give them a community, but we're good people and we are not all witches or warlocks.

But, on the other hand, we do practice magic. Yes, I said it. The elephant in the room has been addressed. That's why you're here after all? Isn't that the lure of the Wiccan faith? Magic? The fact that we acknowledge and believe what everyone in their heart secretly knows that the elements and the forces of the physical and spiritual world are very real and present. Sure, we dabble with primordial forces, but with respect and understanding. No, I cannot turn you into a cat and no I cannot kill you with a spell.

Any true Wicca would rather die than use magic improperly, because there is always a price when it comes to magic.

So, have I piqued your curiosity? Are you interested in knowing more? Then come on in and don't be shy. We'll have a nice little chat and you'll see what it really means to be a Wiccan and I'll tell you about the magic that you know in your heart to be real. I'll give a glimpse at the other side of the world, beyond cell phones and the Internet, where the forests loom and the shadows lurk. There are forces beyond all of us and if you want to know more, I will gladly be your guide.

Concerning Covens:

If you are taking the path that leads you to becoming a Wiccan, you're not like everyone else. You're special, because we do not have Churches, Mosques, or Synagogues on every corner. You will not find temples or university groups, well, you might find a university group or two, but not many. There are a lot of people who like to put on makeup and dress funny and claim to be Wiccans, which makes it hard for newcomers to find a home. If you're serious about becoming a Wiccan or delving into any of the neopagan groups, there are many resources.

Thankfully, we've evolved as a people and the Internet has become a wonderful way for us to connect. After all, Wiccans make up less than one percent of the religious community in America, which makes it hard for our brothers and sisters in Nowhere, Nebraska to commune with us. Thanks to the Internet, there's now a way for us to communicate and encourage one another. It's truly a great tool for us to use.

To read the rest click below!

[Wicca: The Ultimate Beginners Guide For Witches and Warlocks: Learn Wicca Magic Spells, Traditions and Rituals](#)

P.S. You'll find many more books like this and others under my name Michele Gilbert.

Don't miss them… here is a short list.

[Introduction To Palmistry: The Ultimate Palm Reading Guide For Beginners](#)

[Emotional Intelligence: How to Succeed By Mastering Your Emotions And Raising Your IQ](#)

Wicca: The Ultimate Beginners Guide For Witches and Warlocks: Learn Wicca Magic

The Introvert's Advantage: The Introverts Guide To Succeeding In An Extrovert World

Stop Playing Mind Games: How To Free Yourself Of Controlling And Manipulating Relationships

Instant Charisma: A Quick And Easy Guide To Talk, Impress, And Make Anyone Like You

Chakras: Understanding The 7 Main Chakras For Beginners: The Ultimate Guide To Chakra Mindfulness, Balance and Healing

Practicing Mindfulness: Living in the moment through Meditation: Everyday Habits and Rituals to help you achieve inner peace

Adrenal Fatigue: What Is Adrenal Fatigue Syndrome And How To Reset Your Diet And Your Life

[Body Language 101: What A Person's Body Language Is Really Telling You…And How You Can Use It To Your Advantage](#)

Sleep Tight: Overcome Insomnia and Sleep Disorders for a better more restful sleep!

The Arthritis Pain Cure: How to find Arthritis Pain Relief and live a happy pain free life!

The Headache Pain Cure: How to find Headache Pain Relief and live a happy Pain Free Life!

Stop Panic Attacks and Anxiety Disorders without Drugs Now!: Overcome Panic, Stress and Anxiety and live a happy pain free life!

The Breakup Recovery Guide: Advice for Surviving Heartbreak, Letting Go and Thriving in an exciting new life!

The Friendship Guide to Finding Friends Forever: How to Find, Make and Keep Quality Friendships After your Breakup

The Credit Fix: Leave behind credit card debt and poor credit scores and get your life back!

How To Stop Being Jealous And Insecure: Overcome Insecurity And Relationship Jealousy

My Free Gift To You!

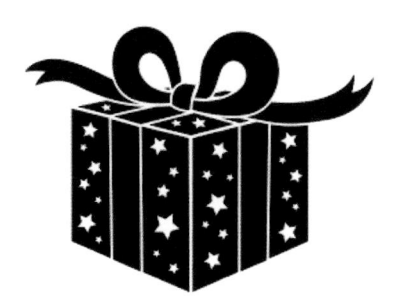

As a way of saying thank you for downloading my book, I am willing to give you access to a selected group of readers who (every week or so) receive inspiring, life-changing kindle books at deep discounts, and sometimes even absolutely free.

Wouldn't it be great to get amazing Kindle offers delivered directly to your inbox?

Wouldn't it be great to be the first to know when I'm releasing new fresh and above all sharply discounted content?

But why would I do something like this?

Why would I offer my books at such a low price and even give them away for free when they took me countless hours to produce?

Simple…. because I want to spread the word.!

For a few short days Amazon allows Kindle authors to promote their newly released books by offering them deeply discounted (up to 70% price discounts and even for free. This allows us to spread the word extremely quickly allowing users to download thousands and thousands of copies in a very short period of time.

Once the timeframe has passed, these books will revert back to their normal selling price. That's why you will benefit from being the first to know when they can be downloaded for free!

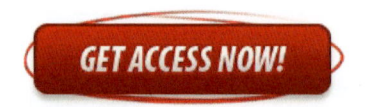

So are you ready to claim your weekly Kindle books?

You are just one click away! Follow the link below and sign up to start receiving awesome content

Thank you and Enjoy!

About Michele

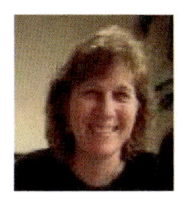

Michele Gilbert was born and raised in Brooklyn, New York. Drawn to literature and writing at a young age, she enrolled at Brooklyn College and majored in English. After graduation Michele did not begin writing immediately, instead she embarked on a career in the finance industry and spent the next thirty years on Wall Street.

Serendipity struck when she least expected it. After ending a long-term relationship, Michele found herself lost and unsure what the future held. She began to read books on grief and loss, looking for answers. Those led her to delve deeper into the Law of Attraction and its power. What resulted was remarkable. Not only had she begun to heal, she had also rekindled her former love of writing and discovered her life's purpose.

The years have taken her through many twists and turns, but she learned valuable lessons along the way. Today she publishes books-mostly self-help and metaphysical in nature-and feels compelled to share her knowledge with those facing similar experiences. Her greatest hope is to inspire others and show them ways to overcome adversity and gracefully accept life's inevitable low points.

Going forward, she plans to incorporate more teachings of self-help, finance and meditation. Regular meditation is very beneficial to her progress as she forges a new life. Morning rituals and positive incantations are other practices Michele embraces; they are very restorative in daily life.

As an avid hiker, Michele and fellow club members often hike the picturesque Jersey Pine Barrens. She is a history buff, voracious reader, baseball fanatic and a foodie. She also proudly supports Trout Unlimited-a national non-profit organization dedicated to conserving, protecting and restoring North America's Coldwater fisheries and their watersheds.

Michele currently resides forty minutes from Atlantic City and the Jersey Shore. She makes her home with a Blue Russian rescue cat named Jersey, though she isn't exactly sure who rescued who.

Michele really enjoys publishing books that can make a difference in people's lives. If you have any suggestions or would like to have a specific topic covered in a future book, please send an email to michelegilbertbooks@gmail.com and we will get back to you.

Thanks for reading!

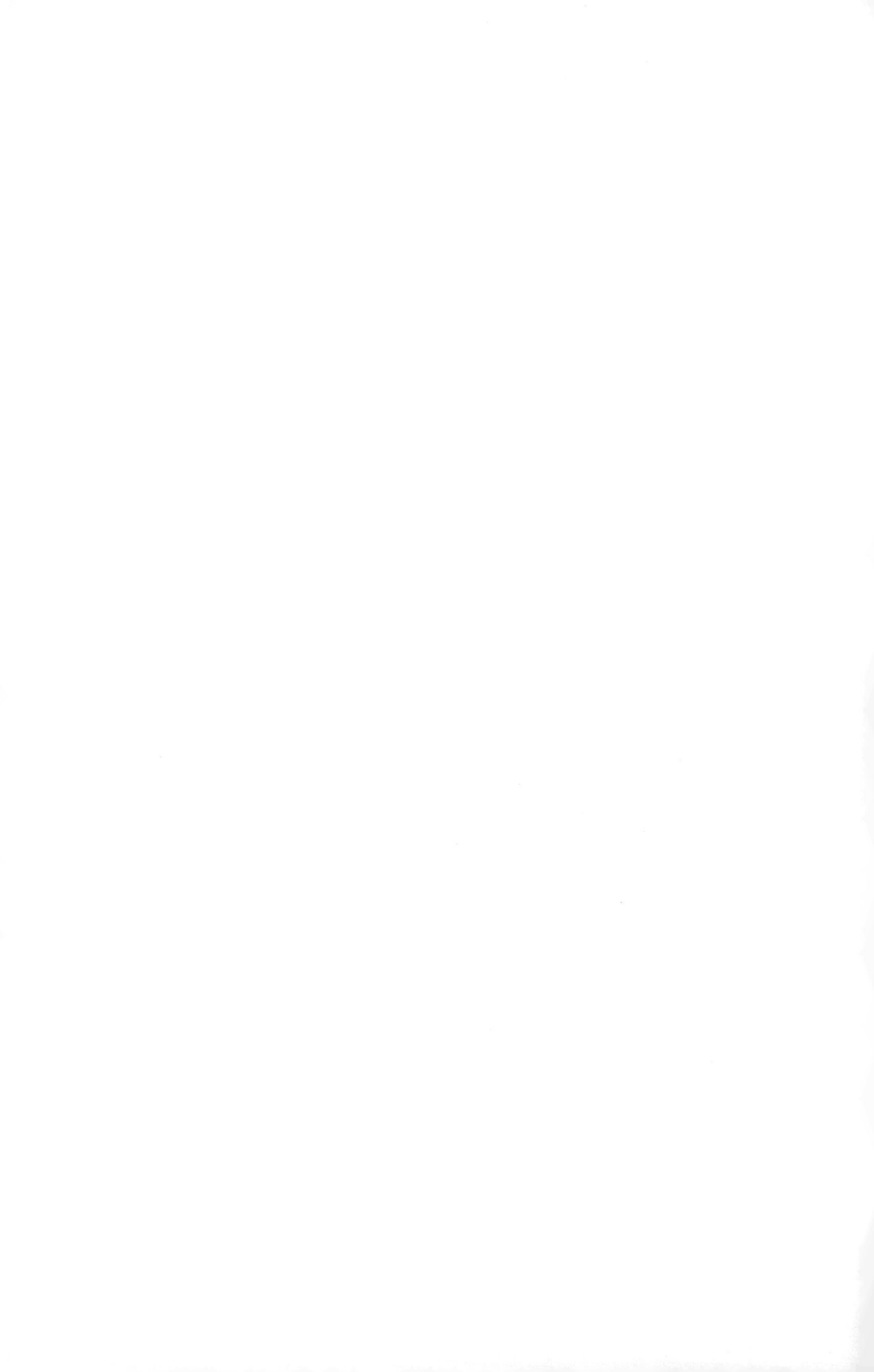

Printed in Great Britain
by Amazon